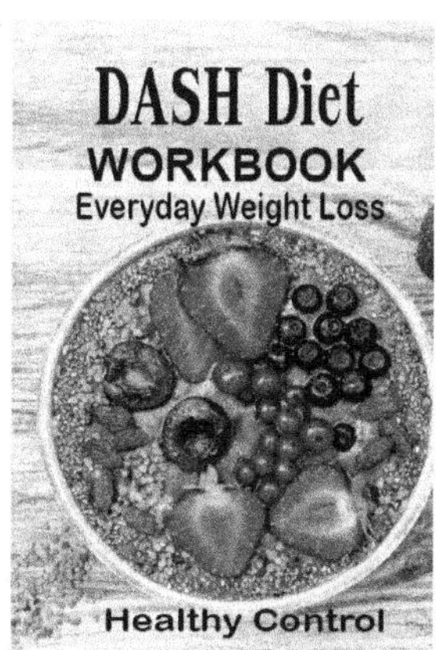

DASH Diet Workbook

Health care is important. In the present we are ill because the

Food we eat incorrectly.,Obesity is the cause of various

Diseases. We need to control eating.,The pattern control is very

Important because we often forget.,Workbook for a Healthy

This Workbook can help you control your eating.And Family

1 Week DASH Diet Workbook..Calories

	Breakfast	Lunch	Dinner	Snacks	DASH Diet
					Base On.............Calories
MONDAY					Note.......................
TUESDAY					Fruits.................. Vegetables...........
WEDNESDAY					Fat free Lowfat Milk dairy.............. Whole Grains ....
THURSDAY					Lean Meat Fish &Poultry............... Nut Seeds & Legumes..............
FRIDAY					Oils..................... .... Sweets Salt.......... .... Alcohol................
SATURDAY					....
SUNDAY					**Gaols Success** Base Planer Calories.................. ....

1 Week DASH Diet Workbook				...................Calories

	Breakfast	Lunch	Dinner	Snacks	DASH Diet Base On............Calories
MONDAY					Note....................... ....
TUESDAY					Fruits................. Vegetables............
WEDNESDAY					Fat free Lowfat Milk dairy.............. Whole Grains ....
THURSDAY					Lean Meat Fish &Poultry............... Nut Seeds & Legumes.............
FRIDAY					Oils...................... .... Sweets Salt.......... Alcohol...............
SATURDAY					....
SUNDAY					Gaols Success Base Planer Calories................. ....

1 Week DASH Diet Workbook...Calories

	Breakfast	Lunch	Dinner	Snacks	DASH Diet
					Base On............Calories
MONDAY					Note........................
TUESDAY					Fruits.................
					Vegetables...........
WEDNESDAY					Fat free Lowfat Milk dairy..............
					Whole Grains
THURSDAY					Lean Meat Fish &Poultry...............
					Nut Seeds & Legumes.............
FRIDAY					Oils......................
					Sweets Salt.......... Alcohol...............
SATURDAY					
SUNDAY					Gaols Success Base Planer Calories..................

1 Week DASH Diet Workbook...Calories

	Breakfast	Lunch	Dinner	Snacks	DASH Diet Base On............Calories
MONDAY					Note........................
TUESDAY					Fruits.................... Vegetables............
WEDNESDAY					Fat free Lowfat Milk dairy.............. Whole Grains
THURSDAY					Lean Meat Fish &Poultry............... Nut Seeds & Legumes..............
FRIDAY					Oils....................... Sweets Salt.......... Alcohol...............
SATURDAY					
SUNDAY					Gaols Success Base Planer Calories..................

1 Week DASH Diet Workbook..Calories

	Breakfast	Lunch	Dinner	Snacks	DASH Diet Base On............Calories
MONDAY					Note.........................
TUESDAY					Fruits.................... Vegetables............
					Fat free Lowfat Milk dairy..............
WEDNESDAY					Whole Grains
THURSDAY					Lean Meat Fish &Poultry............... Nut Seeds & Legumes..............
FRIDAY					Oils....................... Sweets Salt.......... Alcohol...............
SATURDAY					
SUNDAY					Gaols Success Base Planer Calories................

| 1 Week DASH Diet Workbook..Calories | | | | | |

	Breakfast	Lunch	Dinner	Snacks	DASH Diet
					Base On............Calories
MONDAY					Note.......................
TUESDAY					Fruits.................... Vegetables............
					Fat free Lowfat Milk dairy..............
WEDNESDAY					Whole Grains ....
THURSDAY					Lean Meat Fish &Poultry............... Nut Seeds & Legumes..............
FRIDAY					Oils...................... .... Sweets Salt.......... .... Alcohol................
SATURDAY					....
SUNDAY					Gaols Success Base Planer Calories.................. ....

1 Week DASH Diet Workbook..Calories

	Breakfast	Lunch	Dinner	Snacks	DASH Diet
					Base On.............Calories
MONDAY					Note........................
TUESDAY					Fruits................. Vegetables...........
WEDNESDAY					Fat free Lowfat Milk dairy.............. Whole Grains ....
THURSDAY					Lean Meat Fish &Poultry............... Nut Seeds & Legumes..............
FRIDAY					Oils...................... .... Sweets Salt.......... .... Alcohol...............
SATURDAY					
SUNDAY					Gaols Success Base Planer Calories...................

	Breakfast	Lunch	Dinner	Snacks	DASH Diet
					Base On.............Calories
MONDAY					Note........................ ....
TUESDAY					Fruits.................. Vegetables...........
WEDNESDAY					Fat free Lowfat Milk dairy............... Whole Grains ....
THURSDAY					Lean Meat Fish &Poultry............... Nut Seeds & Legumes.............
FRIDAY					Oils..................... .... Sweets Salt.......... .... Alcohol...............
SATURDAY					
SUNDAY					Gaols Success Base Planer Calories................

1 Week DASH Diet Workbook...Calories

1 Week DASH Diet Workbook..Calories

	Breakfast	Lunch	Dinner	Snacks	DASH Diet
					Base On.............Calories
MONDAY					Note........................
TUESDAY					Fruits................... Vegetables............
					Fat free Lowfat Milk dairy..............
WEDNESDAY					Whole Grains ....
THURSDAY					Lean Meat Fish &Poultry............... Nut Seeds & Legumes..............
FRIDAY					Oils....................... .... Sweets Salt.......... .... Alcohol................
SATURDAY					
SUNDAY					Gaols Success Base Planer Calories...................

1 Week DASH Diet Workbook..Calories

	Breakfast	Lunch	Dinner	Snacks	DASH Diet
					Base On.............Calories
MONDAY					Note........................
TUESDAY					Fruits................. Vegetables...........
WEDNESDAY					Fat free Lowfat Milk dairy............. Whole Grains
THURSDAY					Lean Meat Fish &Poultry............... Nut Seeds & Legumes.............
FRIDAY					Oils....................... Sweets Salt.......... Alcohol...............
SATURDAY					
SUNDAY					Gaols Success Base Planer Calories...................

1 Week DASH Diet Workbook...Calories

	Breakfast	Lunch	Dinner	Snacks	DASH Diet
					Base On.............Calories
MONDAY					Note........................
TUESDAY					Fruits................. Vegetables.............
					Fat free Lowfat Milk dairy..............
WEDNESDAY					Whole Grains ....
THURSDAY					Lean Meat Fish &Poultry............... Nut Seeds & Legumes..............
FRIDAY					Oils................ .... Sweets Salt.......... .... Alcohol................
SATURDAY					....
SUNDAY					Gaols Success Base Planer Calories.................... ....

1 Week DASH Diet Workbook...Calories

	Breakfast	Lunch	Dinner	Snacks	DASH Diet Base On............Calories
MONDAY					Note........................ ....
TUESDAY					Fruits.................... Vegetables............
WEDNESDAY					Fat free Lowfat Milk dairy.............. Whole Grains ....
THURSDAY					Lean Meat Fish &Poultry................ Nut Seeds & Legumes..............
FRIDAY					Oils....................... .... Sweets Salt.......... .... Alcohol................
SATURDAY					....
SUNDAY					Gaols Success Base Planer Calories.................... ....

1 Week DASH Diet Workbook..Calories

	Breakfast	Lunch	Dinner	Snacks	DASH Diet Base On............Calories
MONDAY					Note........................
TUESDAY					Fruits................. Vegetables............
WEDNESDAY					Fat free Lowfat Milk dairy.............. Whole Grains
THURSDAY					Lean Meat Fish &Poultry............... Nut Seeds & Legumes.............
FRIDAY					Oils..................... Sweets Salt.......... Alcohol...............
SATURDAY					
SUNDAY					Gaols Success Base Planer Calories...................

1 Week DASH Diet Workbook..Calories

	Breakfast	Lunch	Dinner	Snacks	DASH Diet
					Base On.............Calories
MONDAY					Note......................
TUESDAY					Fruits................... Vegetables............
WEDNESDAY					Fat free Lowfat Milk dairy............... Whole Grains
THURSDAY					Lean Meat Fish &Poultry................ Nut Seeds & Legumes.............
FRIDAY					Oils....................... Sweets Salt.......... Alcohol................
SATURDAY					
SUNDAY					Gaols Success Base Planer Calories..................

	Breakfast	Lunch	Dinner	Snacks	DASH Diet
					Base On.............Calories
MONDAY					Note..................... ....
TUESDAY					Fruits.................... Vegetables............
					Fat free Lowfat Milk dairy...............
WEDNESDAY					Whole Grains ....
THURSDAY					Lean Meat Fish &Poultry................ Nut Seeds & Legumes...............
FRIDAY					Oils....................... .... Sweets Salt.......... .... Alcohol.................
SATURDAY					.... **Gaols Success** Base Planer
SUNDAY					Calories.................... ....

1 Week DASH Diet Workbook...Calories

	Breakfast	Lunch	Dinner	Snacks	DASH Diet Base On............Calories
MONDAY					Note........................
TUESDAY					Fruits................ Vegetables............
WEDNESDAY					Fat free Lowfat Milk dairy..............
					Whole Grains
THURSDAY					Lean Meat Fish &Poultry................ Nut Seeds & Legumes..............
FRIDAY					Oils...................... Sweets Salt.......... Alcohol................
SATURDAY					
SUNDAY					Gaols Success Base Planer Calories...................

| 1 Week DASH Diet Workbook..Calories | | | | |
| | | | | |

	Breakfast	Lunch	Dinner	Snacks	DASH Diet Base On............Calories
MONDAY					Note........................
TUESDAY					Fruits.................... Vegetables............
					Fat free Lowfat Milk dairy...............
WEDNESDAY					Whole Grains ....
THURSDAY					Lean Meat Fish &Poultry................ Nut Seeds & Legumes..............
FRIDAY					Oils....................... .... Sweets Salt.......... .... Alcohol................
SATURDAY					....
SUNDAY					Gaols Success Base Planer Calories................... ....

1 Week DASH Diet Workbook..Calories				

	Breakfast	Lunch	Dinner	Snacks	DASH Diet
					Base On..............Calories
MONDAY					Note........................ ....
TUESDAY					Fruits................. Vegetables............
					Fat free Lowfat Milk dairy..............
WEDNESDAY					Whole Grains ....
THURSDAY					Lean Meat Fish &Poultry............... Nut Seeds & Legumes..............
FRIDAY					Oils...................... .... Sweets Salt.......... Alcohol................
SATURDAY					.... Gaols Success Base Planer
SUNDAY					Calories................. ....

1 Week DASH Diet Workbook...Calories				

	Breakfast	Lunch	Dinner	Snacks	DASH Diet Base On............Calories
MONDAY					Note........................
TUESDAY					Fruits................... Vegetables............ Fat free Lowfat Milk dairy..............
WEDNESDAY					Whole Grains ....
THURSDAY					Lean Meat Fish &Poultry................ Nut Seeds & Legumes..............
FRIDAY					Oils...................... .... Sweets Salt.......... Alcohol...............
SATURDAY					....
SUNDAY					Gaols Success Base Planer Calories................... ....

1 Week DASH Diet Workbook..Calories

	Breakfast	Lunch	Dinner	Snacks	DASH Diet Base On............Calories
MONDAY					Note....................... ....
TUESDAY					Fruits................... Vegetables............
WEDNESDAY					Fat free Lowfat Milk dairy.............. Whole Grains ....
THURSDAY					Lean Meat Fish &Poultry................ Nut Seeds & Legumes...............
FRIDAY					Oils....................... .... Sweets Salt.......... ..... Alcohol.................
SATURDAY					....
SUNDAY					Gaols Success Base Planer Calories................... ....

1 Week DASH Diet Workbook..Calories

	Breakfast	Lunch	Dinner	Snacks	DASH Diet Base On.............Calories
MONDAY					Note......................... ....
TUESDAY					Fruits................... Vegetables............
WEDNESDAY					Fat free Lowfat Milk dairy.............. Whole Grains ....
THURSDAY					Lean Meat Fish &Poultry............... Nut Seeds & Legumes.............
FRIDAY					Oils..................... .... Sweets Salt.......... .... Alcohol................
SATURDAY					....
SUNDAY					Gaols Success Base Planer Calories................... ....

1 Week DASH Diet Workbook..Calories					
	Breakfast	**Lunch**	**Dinner**	**Snacks**	**DASH Diet** Base On............Calories
MONDAY					Note........................
TUESDAY					Fruits.................. Vegetables...........
WEDNESDAY					Fat free Lowfat Milk dairy.............. / Whole Grains
THURSDAY					Lean Meat Fish &Poultry............... / Nut Seeds & Legumes..............
FRIDAY					Oils...................... / Sweets Salt.......... Alcohol...............
SATURDAY					Gaols Success Base Planer Calories...................
SUNDAY					

1 Week DASH Diet Workbook...Calories

	Breakfast	Lunch	Dinner	Snacks	DASH Diet
					Base On...........Calories
MONDAY					Note........................
TUESDAY					Fruits................. Vegetables...........
					Fat free Lowfat Milk dairy..............
WEDNESDAY					Whole Grains ....
THURSDAY					Lean Meat Fish &Poultry...............
					Nut Seeds & Legumes..............
FRIDAY					Oils...................... ....
					Sweets Salt.......... Alcohol...............
SATURDAY					
					Gaols Success Base Planer Calories..................
SUNDAY					

1 Week DASH Diet Workbook...Calories

	Breakfast	Lunch	Dinner	Snacks	DASH Diet Base On.............Calories
MONDAY					Note........................ ....
TUESDAY					Fruits................. Vegetables.............
WEDNESDAY					Fat free Lowfat Milk dairy..............
					Whole Grains ....
THURSDAY					Lean Meat Fish &Poultry................
					Nut Seeds & Legumes..............
FRIDAY					Oils........................ ....
					Sweets Salt.......... Alcohol................
SATURDAY					
SUNDAY					Gaols Success Base Planer Calories..................

1 Week DASH Diet Workbook..Calories

	Breakfast	Lunch	Dinner	Snacks	DASH Diet
					Base On............Calories
MONDAY					Note........................
TUESDAY					Fruits.................. Vegetables...........
WEDNESDAY					Fat free Lowfat Milk dairy.............. Whole Grains
THURSDAY					Lean Meat Fish &Poultry............. Nut Seeds & Legumes.............
FRIDAY					Oils...................... Sweets Salt.......... Alcohol...............
SATURDAY					Gaols Success Base Planer Calories..................
SUNDAY					

1 Week DASH Diet Workbook...Calories

	Breakfast	Lunch	Dinner	Snacks	DASH Diet Base On.............Calories
MONDAY					Note...................... ....
TUESDAY					Fruits................. Vegetables............
WEDNESDAY					Fat free Lowfat Milk dairy.............. Whole Grains ....
THURSDAY					Lean Meat Fish &Poultry................ Nut Seeds & Legumes...............
FRIDAY					Oils....................... .... Sweets Salt.......... .... Alcohol................
SATURDAY					....
SUNDAY					Gaols Success Base Planer Calories................... ....

1 Week DASH Diet Workbook..Calories				
	Breakfast	Lunch	Dinner	Snacks	DASH Diet Base On.............Calories
MONDAY					Note........................
TUESDAY					Fruits.................... Vegetables.............
WEDNESDAY					Fat free Lowfat Milk dairy............... Whole Grains
THURSDAY					Lean Meat Fish &Poultry................ Nut Seeds & Legumes..............
FRIDAY					Oils...................... Sweets Salt.......... Alcohol................
SATURDAY					
SUNDAY					Gaols Success Base Planer Calories...................

1 Week DASH Diet Workbook..Calories				
	Breakfast	**Lunch**	**Dinner**	**Snacks**	**DASH Diet** Base On.............Calories

	Breakfast	Lunch	Dinner	Snacks	DASH Diet Base On.............Calories
MONDAY					Note...................... ....
TUESDAY					Fruits.................. Vegetables...........
WEDNESDAY					Fat free Lowfat Milk dairy.............. Whole Grains ....
THURSDAY					Lean Meat Fish &Poultry................ Nut Seeds & Legumes..............
FRIDAY					Oils....................... .... Sweets Salt.......... .... Alcohol................
SATURDAY					....
SUNDAY					**Gaols Success** Base Planer Calories................... ....

1 Week DASH Diet Workbook...Calories

	Breakfast	Lunch	Dinner	Snacks	DASH Diet Base On............Calories
MONDAY					Note.........................
TUESDAY					Fruits................... Vegetables............
WEDNESDAY					Fat free Lowfat Milk dairy............... Whole Grains ....
THURSDAY					Lean Meat Fish &Poultry................ Nut Seeds & Legumes.............
FRIDAY					Oils........................ .... Sweets Salt.......... .... Alcohol................
SATURDAY					....
SUNDAY					Gaols Success Base Planer Calories................. ....

1 Week DASH Diet Workbook......................................Calories

	Breakfast	Lunch	Dinner	Snacks	DASH Diet
					Base On.............Calories
MONDAY					Note......................
TUESDAY					Fruits................... Vegetables............
					Fat free Lowfat Milk dairy..............
WEDNESDAY					Whole Grains ....
THURSDAY					Lean Meat Fish &Poultry............... Nut Seeds & Legumes..............
FRIDAY					Oils...................... .... Sweets Salt.......... .... Alcohol................
SATURDAY					
SUNDAY					Gaols Success Base Planer Calories....................

1 Week DASH Diet Workbook...Calories

	Breakfast	Lunch	Dinner	Snacks	DASH Diet
					Base On.............Calories
MONDAY					Note.........................
TUESDAY					Fruits.................. Vegetables............
WEDNESDAY					Fat free Lowfat Milk dairy.............. Whole Grains ....
THURSDAY					Lean Meat Fish &Poultry............... Nut Seeds & Legumes..............
FRIDAY					Oils...................... Sweets Salt.......... Alcohol................
SATURDAY					
SUNDAY					Gaols Success Base Planer Calories.................

1 Week DASH Diet Workbook..Calories

	Breakfast	Lunch	Dinner	Snacks	DASH Diet Base On............Calories
MONDAY					Note........................ ....
TUESDAY					Fruits.................. Vegetables............
WEDNESDAY					Fat free Lowfat Milk dairy.............. Whole Grains ....
THURSDAY					Lean Meat Fish &Poultry............... Nut Seeds & Legumes..............
FRIDAY					Oils...................... .... Sweets Salt.......... .... Alcohol................
SATURDAY					....
SUNDAY					Gaols Success Base Planer Calories................... ....

	Breakfast	Lunch	Dinner	Snacks	DASH Diet
					Base On.............Calories
MONDAY					Note....................
TUESDAY					Fruits................. Vegetables............
WEDNESDAY					Fat free Lowfat Milk dairy.............. Whole Grains
THURSDAY					Lean Meat Fish &Poultry............... Nut Seeds & Legumes.............
FRIDAY					Oils.................... Sweets Salt.......... Alcohol................
SATURDAY					
SUNDAY					Gaols Success Base Planer Calories................

1 Week DASH Diet Workbook...Calories

1 Week DASH Diet Workbook...Calories					
	Breakfast	**Lunch**	**Dinner**	**Snacks**	**DASH Diet** Base On............Calories
MONDAY					Note....................... ....
TUESDAY					Fruits................. Vegetables...........
					Fat free Lowfat Milk dairy.............
WEDNESDAY					Whole Grains ....
THURSDAY					Lean Meat Fish &Poultry............... Nut Seeds & Legumes..............
FRIDAY					Oils...................... .... Sweets Salt.......... .... Alcohol................
SATURDAY					....
SUNDAY					**Gaols Success** Base Planer Calories................... ....

1 Week DASH Diet Workbook...Calories

	Breakfast	Lunch	Dinner	Snacks	DASH Diet Base On.............Calories
MONDAY					Note........................ ....
TUESDAY					Fruits................... Vegetables............
WEDNESDAY					Fat free Lowfat Milk dairy.............. Whole Grains ....
THURSDAY					Lean Meat Fish &Poultry................ Nut Seeds & Legumes.............
FRIDAY					Oils...................... .... Sweets Salt.......... ...... Alcohol................
SATURDAY					....
SUNDAY					**Gaols Success** Base Planer Calories.................... ....

1 Week DASH Diet Workbook..Calories					

	Breakfast	Lunch	Dinner	Snacks	DASH Diet Base On.............Calories
MONDAY					Note........................ ....
TUESDAY					Fruits................... Vegetables............
WEDNESDAY					Fat free Lowfat Milk dairy.............. Whole Grains ....
THURSDAY					Lean Meat Fish &Poultry................ Nut Seeds & Legumes..............
FRIDAY					Oils...................... .... Sweets Salt.......... .... Alcohol................
SATURDAY					....
SUNDAY					Gaols Success Base Planer Calories.................... ....

1 Week DASH Diet Workbook...Calories

	Breakfast	Lunch	Dinner	Snacks	DASH Diet Base On............Calories
MONDAY					Note....................... ....
TUESDAY					Fruits................... Vegetables............
WEDNESDAY					Fat free Lowfat Milk dairy............. Whole Grains ....
THURSDAY					Lean Meat Fish &Poultry............... Nut Seeds & Legumes...............
FRIDAY					Oils....................... .... Sweets Salt.......... .... Alcohol................
SATURDAY					.... **Gaols Success** Base Planer
SUNDAY					Calories.................. ....

1 Week DASH Diet Workbook..Calories				

	Breakfast	Lunch	Dinner	Snacks	DASH Diet Base On.............Calories
MONDAY					Note........................ ....
TUESDAY					Fruits................... Vegetables............
WEDNESDAY					Fat free Lowfat Milk dairy............... Whole Grains ....
THURSDAY					Lean Meat Fish &Poultry................ Nut Seeds & Legumes..............
FRIDAY					Oils....................... .... Sweets Salt.......... .... Alcohol................
SATURDAY					....
SUNDAY					Gaols Success Base Planer Calories.................. ....

1 Week DASH Diet Workbook...Calories

	Breakfast	Lunch	Dinner	Snacks	DASH Diet
					Base On.............Calories
MONDAY					Note.................... ....
TUESDAY					Fruits.................. Vegetables............
					Fat free Lowfat Milk dairy...............
WEDNESDAY					Whole Grains ....
THURSDAY					Lean Meat Fish &Poultry...............
					Nut Seeds & Legumes...............
FRIDAY					Oils..................... ....
					Sweets Salt........... .... Alcohol.................
SATURDAY					....
SUNDAY					Gaols Success Base Planer Calories................. ....

1 Week DASH Diet Workbook..Calories					
	Breakfast	**Lunch**	**Dinner**	**Snacks**	**DASH Diet** Base On............Calories
MONDAY					Note........................ Fruits.................... Vegetables............
TUESDAY					
WEDNESDAY					Fat free Lowfat Milk dairy.............. Whole Grains ....
THURSDAY					Lean Meat Fish &Poultry............... Nut Seeds & Legumes..............
FRIDAY					Oils...................... .... Sweets Salt.......... Alcohol...............
SATURDAY					
SUNDAY					**Gaols Success** Base Planer Calories...................

1 Week DASH Diet Workbook...Calories

	Breakfast	Lunch	Dinner	Snacks	DASH Diet
					Base On.............Calories
MONDAY					Note........................
TUESDAY					Fruits................. Vegetables............
					Fat free Lowfat Milk dairy..............
WEDNESDAY					Whole Grains ....
THURSDAY					Lean Meat Fish &Poultry................
					Nut Seeds & Legumes..............
FRIDAY					Oils..................... ....
					Sweets Salt.......... Alcohol...............
SATURDAY					
					Gaols Success Base Planer Calories...................
SUNDAY					

1 Week DASH Diet Workbook..Calories

	Breakfast	Lunch	Dinner	Snacks	DASH Diet Base On............Calories
MONDAY					Note......................
TUESDAY					Fruits................... Vegetables............
WEDNESDAY					Fat free Lowfat Milk dairy.............. Whole Grains ....
THURSDAY					Lean Meat Fish &Poultry................ Nut Seeds & Legumes...............
FRIDAY					Oils...................... .... Sweets Salt.......... .... Alcohol................
SATURDAY					....
SUNDAY					Gaols Success Base Planer Calories.................... ....

1 Week DASH Diet Workbook...Calories

	Breakfast	Lunch	Dinner	Snacks	DASH Diet
					Base On.............Calories
MONDAY					Note........................
TUESDAY					Fruits................. Vegetables...........
					Fat free Lowfat Milk dairy.............
WEDNESDAY					Whole Grains
THURSDAY					Lean Meat Fish &Poultry...............
					Nut Seeds & Legumes.............
FRIDAY					Oils......................
					Sweets Salt.......... Alcohol................
SATURDAY					
SUNDAY					Gaols Success Base Planer Calories..................

1 Week DASH Diet Workbook...Calories

	Breakfast	Lunch	Dinner	Snacks	DASH Diet Base On.............Calories
MONDAY					Note........................
TUESDAY					Fruits................. Vegetables...........
WEDNESDAY					Fat free Lowfat Milk dairy............. Whole Grains
THURSDAY					Lean Meat Fish &Poultry............... Nut Seeds & Legumes..............
FRIDAY					Oils...................... Sweets Salt.......... Alcohol................
SATURDAY					
SUNDAY					Gaols Success Base Planer Calories..................

1 Week DASH Diet Workbook...Calories

	Breakfast	Lunch	Dinner	Snacks	DASH Diet
MONDAY					Base On.............Calories Note........................
TUESDAY					Fruits................... Vegetables............
WEDNESDAY					Fat free Lowfat Milk dairy............... Whole Grains ....
THURSDAY					Lean Meat Fish &Poultry............... Nut Seeds & Legumes.............
FRIDAY					Oils....................... .... Sweets Salt.......... .... Alcohol................
SATURDAY					....
SUNDAY					Gaols Success Base Planer Calories................... ....

1 Week DASH Diet Workbook..Calories

	Breakfast	Lunch	Dinner	Snacks	DASH Diet Base On............Calories
MONDAY					Note......................
TUESDAY					Fruits................. Vegetables............
WEDNESDAY					Fat free Lowfat Milk dairy..............
THURSDAY					Whole Grains Lean Meat Fish &Poultry............... Nut Seeds & Legumes..............
FRIDAY					Oils...................... Sweets Salt.......... Alcohol...............
SATURDAY					
SUNDAY					Gaols Success Base Planer Calories....................

	Breakfast	**Lunch**	**Dinner**	**Snacks**	**DASH Diet** Base On............Calories
MONDAY					Note......................
TUESDAY					Fruits................... Vegetables...........
WEDNESDAY					Fat free Lowfat Milk dairy............... Whole Grains
THURSDAY					Lean Meat Fish &Poultry............... Nut Seeds & Legumes...............
FRIDAY					Oils...................... Sweets Salt.......... Alcohol................
SATURDAY					
SUNDAY					**Gaols Success** Base Planer Calories...................

1 Week DASH Diet Workbook...Calories

1 Week DASH Diet Workbook...Calories

	Breakfast	Lunch	Dinner	Snacks	DASH Diet
					Base On.............Calories
MONDAY					Note.........................
TUESDAY					Fruits................... Vegetables.............
					Fat free Lowfat Milk dairy..............
WEDNESDAY					Whole Grains
THURSDAY					Lean Meat Fish &Poultry................
					Nut Seeds & Legumes..............
FRIDAY					Oils......................
					Sweets Salt.......... Alcohol................
SATURDAY					
SUNDAY					Gaols Success Base Planer Calories...................

1 Week DASH Diet Workbook..Calories

	Breakfast	Lunch	Dinner	Snacks	DASH Diet
MONDAY					
TUESDAY					
WEDNESDAY					
THURSDAY					
FRIDAY					
SATURDAY					
SUNDAY					

DASH Diet

Base On.............Calories

Note.........................

Fruits...................
Vegetables............

Fat free Lowfat
Milk dairy...............

Whole Grains
....

Lean Meat Fish
&Poultry...............

Nut Seeds
& Legumes.............

Oils........................
....
....

Sweets Salt...........
...
Alcohol................

Gaols Success

Base Planer

Calories....................

1 Week DASH Diet Workbook..Calories

	Breakfast	Lunch	Dinner	Snacks	DASH Diet
					Base On.............Calories
MONDAY					Note......................... ....
TUESDAY					Fruits................... Vegetables............
					Fat free Lowfat Milk dairy..............
WEDNESDAY					Whole Grains ....
THURSDAY					Lean Meat Fish &Poultry................
					Nut Seeds & Legumes...............
FRIDAY					Oils....................... ....
					Sweets Salt.......... .... Alcohol.................
SATURDAY					....
SUNDAY					Gaols Success Base Planer Calories.................... ....

1 Week DASH Diet Workbook...Calories

	Breakfast	Lunch	Dinner	Snacks	DASH Diet Base On.............Calories
MONDAY					Note........................
TUESDAY					Fruits.................. Vegetables...........
WEDNESDAY					Fat free Lowfat Milk dairy.............. Whole Grains ....
THURSDAY					Lean Meat Fish &Poultry............... Nut Seeds & Legumes..............
FRIDAY					Oils....................... .... Sweets Salt.......... .... Alcohol................
SATURDAY					.... Gaols Success Base Planer
SUNDAY					Calories................... ....

1 Week DASH Diet Workbook..Calories

	Breakfast	Lunch	Dinner	Snacks	DASH Diet Base On.............Calories
MONDAY					Note.........................
TUESDAY					Fruits.................... Vegetables...........
WEDNESDAY					Fat free Lowfat Milk dairy.............. Whole Grains
THURSDAY					Lean Meat Fish &Poultry............... Nut Seeds & Legumes..............
FRIDAY					Oils...................... Sweets Salt......... Alcohol...............
SATURDAY					
SUNDAY					Gaols Success Base Planer Calories..................

1 Week DASH Diet Workbook...Calories

	Breakfast	Lunch	Dinner	Snacks	DASH Diet
					Base On............Calories
MONDAY					Note.......................
TUESDAY					Fruits................. Vegetables............
					Fat free Lowfat Milk dairy..............
WEDNESDAY					Whole Grains ....
THURSDAY					Lean Meat Fish &Poultry............... Nut Seeds & Legumes..............
FRIDAY					Oils....................... .... Sweets Salt.......... .... Alcohol................
SATURDAY					....
SUNDAY					Gaols Success Base Planer Calories................... ....

1 Week DASH Diet Workbook...Calories				

	Breakfast	Lunch	Dinner	Snacks	DASH Diet Base On............Calories
MONDAY					Note........................
TUESDAY					Fruits.................... Vegetables............
					Fat free Lowfat Milk dairy..............
WEDNESDAY					Whole Grains ....
THURSDAY					Lean Meat Fish &Poultry................ Nut Seeds & Legumes..............
FRIDAY					Oils...................... .... Sweets Salt.......... .... Alcohol................
SATURDAY					....
SUNDAY					Gaols Success Base Planer Calories................... ....

1 Week DASH Diet Workbook...Calories

	Breakfast	Lunch	Dinner	Snacks	DASH Diet
					Base On............Calories
MONDAY					Note........................
TUESDAY					Fruits................... Vegetables............
					Fat free Lowfat Milk dairy..............
WEDNESDAY					Whole Grains
THURSDAY					Lean Meat Fish &Poultry................ Nut Seeds & Legumes..............
FRIDAY					Oils...................... Sweets Salt.......... Alcohol...............
SATURDAY					
SUNDAY					Gaols Success Base Planer Calories..................

1 Week DASH Diet Workbook...Calories

	Breakfast	Lunch	Dinner	Snacks	DASH Diet
					Base On.............Calories
MONDAY					Note........................
TUESDAY					Fruits................... Vegetables...........
WEDNESDAY					Fat free Lowfat Milk dairy............... Whole Grains
THURSDAY					Lean Meat Fish &Poultry................ Nut Seeds & Legumes.............
FRIDAY					Oils...................... Sweets Salt.......... Alcohol................
SATURDAY					
SUNDAY					Gaols Success Base Planer Calories...................

1 Week DASH Diet Workbook...Calories

	Breakfast	Lunch	Dinner	Snacks	DASH Diet
					Base On.............Calories
MONDAY					Note........................
TUESDAY					Fruits................... Vegetables.............
WEDNESDAY					Fat free Lowfat Milk dairy............... Whole Grains
THURSDAY					Lean Meat Fish &Poultry............... Nut Seeds & Legumes..............
FRIDAY					Oils....................... Sweets Salt.......... Alcohol................
SATURDAY					
SUNDAY					**Gaols Success** Base Planer Calories....................

1 Week DASH Diet Workbook..Calories

	Breakfast	Lunch	Dinner	Snacks	DASH Diet
MONDAY					Base On............Calories Note........................
TUESDAY					Fruits..................... Vegetables............ Fat free Lowfat Milk dairy..............
WEDNESDAY					Whole Grains
THURSDAY					Lean Meat Fish &Poultry............... Nut Seeds & Legumes..............
FRIDAY					Oils....................... Sweets Salt.......... Alcohol................
SATURDAY					Gaols Success Base Planer
SUNDAY					Calories....................

1 Week DASH Diet Workbook...Calories

	Breakfast	Lunch	Dinner	Snacks	DASH Diet
					Base On............Calories
MONDAY					Note....................... ....
TUESDAY					.... Fruits................... Vegetables............
WEDNESDAY					Fat free Lowfat Milk dairy.............. Whole Grains ....
THURSDAY					Lean Meat Fish &Poultry................ Nut Seeds & Legumes...............
FRIDAY					Oils....................... .... Sweets Salt........... .... Alcohol..................
SATURDAY					....
SUNDAY					Gaols Success Base Planer Calories................... ....

1 Week DASH Diet Workbook..Calories

	Breakfast	Lunch	Dinner	Snacks	DASH Diet
					Base On.............Calories
					Note........................
MONDAY					
TUESDAY					Fruits..................
					Vegetables............
					Fat free Lowfat Milk dairy..............
WEDNESDAY					Whole Grains
THURSDAY					Lean Meat Fish &Poultry...............
					Nut Seeds & Legumes..............
FRIDAY					Oils......................
					Sweets Salt.......... Alcohol...............
SATURDAY					
SUNDAY					Gaols Success Base Planer Calories..................

1 Week DASH Diet Workbook..Calories

	Breakfast	Lunch	Dinner	Snacks	DASH Diet
					Base On.............Calories
MONDAY					Note.........................
TUESDAY					Fruits.................... Vegetables............
					Fat free Lowfat Milk dairy..............
WEDNESDAY					Whole Grains ....
THURSDAY					Lean Meat Fish &Poultry............... Nut Seeds & Legumes.............
FRIDAY					Oils..................... .... Sweets Salt.......... Alcohol...............
SATURDAY					Gaols Success Base Planer Calories...................
SUNDAY					

1 Week DASH Diet Workbook..Calories				

	Breakfast	Lunch	Dinner	Snacks	DASH Diet Base On............Calories
MONDAY					Note...................... ....
TUESDAY					Fruits................. Vegetables............
WEDNESDAY					Fat free Lowfat Milk dairy............... Whole Grains ....
THURSDAY					Lean Meat Fish &Poultry............... Nut Seeds & Legumes...............
FRIDAY					Oils..................... .... Sweets Salt.......... Alcohol................
SATURDAY					....
SUNDAY					Gaols Success Base Planer Calories................... ....

1 Week DASH Diet Workbook...Calories

	Breakfast	Lunch	Dinner	Snacks	DASH Diet Base On.............Calories
MONDAY					Note........................
TUESDAY					Fruits.................. Vegetables............
					Fat free Lowfat Milk dairy..............
WEDNESDAY					Whole Grains ....
THURSDAY					Lean Meat Fish &Poultry.............. Nut Seeds & Legumes.............
FRIDAY					Oils...................... Sweets Salt.......... Alcohol...............
SATURDAY					
SUNDAY					Gaols Success Base Planer Calories...................

1 Week DASH Diet Workbook...Calories

	Breakfast	Lunch	Dinner	Snacks	DASH Diet
MONDAY					Base On.............Calories
					Note.......................
TUESDAY					Fruits................... / Vegetables............
WEDNESDAY					Fat free Lowfat Milk dairy.............. / Whole Grains
THURSDAY					Lean Meat Fish &Poultry............... / Nut Seeds & Legumes..............
FRIDAY					Oils....................... / Sweets Salt.......... / Alcohol................
SATURDAY					Gaols Success Base Planer Calories..................
SUNDAY					

1 Week DASH Diet Workbook..Calories

	Breakfast	Lunch	Dinner	Snacks	DASH Diet Base On............Calories
MONDAY					Note........................
TUESDAY					Fruits................. Vegetables............
WEDNESDAY					Fat free Lowfat Milk dairy............... Whole Grains
THURSDAY					Lean Meat Fish &Poultry................ Nut Seeds & Legumes...............
FRIDAY					Oils...................... Sweets Salt.......... Alcohol...............
SATURDAY					
SUNDAY					Gaols Success Base Planer Calories...................

1 Week DASH Diet Workbook..Calories

	Breakfast	Lunch	Dinner	Snacks	DASH Diet
					Base On............Calories
MONDAY					Note........................
TUESDAY					Fruits..................
					Vegetables............
WEDNESDAY					Fat free Lowfat Milk dairy..............
					Whole Grains
THURSDAY					Lean Meat Fish &Poultry...............
					Nut Seeds & Legumes..............
FRIDAY					Oils......................
					Sweets Salt.......... Alcohol...............
SATURDAY					
SUNDAY					Gaols Success Base Planer Calories..................

1 Week DASH Diet Workbook..Calories					
	Breakfast	**Lunch**	**Dinner**	**Snacks**	**DASH Diet** Base On............Calories
MONDAY					Note......................
TUESDAY					Fruits................. Vegetables...........
WEDNESDAY					Fat free Lowfat Milk dairy.............. Whole Grains
THURSDAY					Lean Meat Fish &Poultry............... Nut Seeds & Legumes..............
FRIDAY					Oils..................... Sweets Salt.......... Alcohol...............
SATURDAY					
SUNDAY					Gaols Success Base Planer Calories....................

1 Week DASH Diet Workbook..Calories				

	Breakfast	Lunch	Dinner	Snacks	DASH Diet Base On.............Calories
MONDAY					Note....................... ....
TUESDAY					Fruits.................. Vegetables...........
WEDNESDAY					Fat free Lowfat Milk dairy.............. Whole Grains ....
THURSDAY					Lean Meat Fish &Poultry................ Nut Seeds & Legumes..............
FRIDAY					Oils....................... .... Sweets Salt.......... .... Alcohol................
SATURDAY					....
SUNDAY					Gaols Success Base Planer Calories................... ....

1 Week DASH Diet Workbook...Calories

	Breakfast	Lunch	Dinner	Snacks	DASH Diet
					Base On.............Calories
MONDAY					Note.....................
TUESDAY					Fruits................. Vegetables............
					Fat free Lowfat Milk dairy..............
WEDNESDAY					Whole Grains ....
THURSDAY					Lean Meat Fish &Poultry............... Nut Seeds & Legumes..............
FRIDAY					Oils.................... .... Sweets Salt......... ...... Alcohol................
SATURDAY					
SUNDAY					Gaols Success Base Planer Calories...................

1 Week DASH Diet Workbook...Calories

	Breakfast	Lunch	Dinner	Snacks	DASH Diet Base On............Calories
MONDAY					Note....................... ....
TUESDAY					Fruits................. Vegetables............
WEDNESDAY					Fat free Lowfat Milk dairy.............. Whole Grains ....
THURSDAY					Lean Meat Fish &Poultry............... Nut Seeds & Legumes..............
FRIDAY					Oils....................... .... Sweets Salt.......... Alcohol................
SATURDAY					....
SUNDAY					Gaols Success Base Planer Calories................... ....

1 Week DASH Diet Workbook..Calories

	Breakfast	Lunch	Dinner	Snacks	DASH Diet Base On............Calories
MONDAY					Note.........................
TUESDAY					Fruits.................... Vegetables............
					Fat free Lowfat Milk dairy..............
WEDNESDAY					Whole Grains
THURSDAY					Lean Meat Fish &Poultry................ Nut Seeds & Legumes..............
FRIDAY					Oils...................... Sweets Salt.......... Alcohol................
SATURDAY					
SUNDAY					Gaols Success Base Planer Calories.................

1 Week DASH Diet Workbook...Calories

	Breakfast	Lunch	Dinner	Snacks	DASH Diet
					Base On............Calories
MONDAY					Note........................
TUESDAY					Fruits................. Vegetables............
WEDNESDAY					Fat free Lowfat Milk dairy.............. Whole Grains
THURSDAY					Lean Meat Fish &Poultry............... Nut Seeds & Legumes..............
FRIDAY					Oils...................... Sweets Salt.......... Alcohol...............
SATURDAY					
SUNDAY					Gaols Success Base Planer Calories..................

1 Week DASH Diet Workbook...Calories

	Breakfast	Lunch	Dinner	Snacks	DASH Diet
					Base On............Calories
MONDAY					Note........................
TUESDAY					Fruits................. Vegetables...........
WEDNESDAY					Fat free Lowfat Milk dairy.............. Whole Grains
THURSDAY					Lean Meat Fish &Poultry............... Nut Seeds & Legumes.............
FRIDAY					Oils..................... Sweets Salt.......... Alcohol...............
SATURDAY					Gaols Success Base Planer Calories..................
SUNDAY					

<table>
<tr><td colspan="6">1 Week DASH Diet Workbook...Calories</td></tr>
<tr><td></td><td>Breakfast</td><td>Lunch</td><td>Dinner</td><td>Snacks</td><td>DASH Diet
Base On.............Calories</td></tr>
<tr><td>MONDAY</td><td></td><td></td><td></td><td></td><td>Note........................
....
....
....
....
....
....
....
...................................</td></tr>
<tr><td>TUESDAY</td><td></td><td></td><td></td><td></td><td>Fruits...................
Vegetables...........</td></tr>
<tr><td>WEDNESDAY</td><td></td><td></td><td></td><td></td><td>Fat free Lowfat
Milk dairy..............

Whole Grains
............................</td></tr>
<tr><td>THURSDAY</td><td></td><td></td><td></td><td></td><td>Lean Meat Fish
&Poultry...............

Nut Seeds
& Legumes.............</td></tr>
<tr><td>FRIDAY</td><td></td><td></td><td></td><td></td><td>Oils......................
....
....

Sweets Salt..........
....
Alcohol...............</td></tr>
<tr><td>SATURDAY</td><td></td><td></td><td></td><td></td><td>............................
....
............................</td></tr>
<tr><td>SUNDAY</td><td></td><td></td><td></td><td></td><td>Gaols Success
Base Planer
Calories...................
....
............................</td></tr>
</table>

1 Week DASH Diet Workbook...Calories

	Breakfast	Lunch	Dinner	Snacks	DASH Diet Base On............Calories
MONDAY					Note......................................
TUESDAY					Fruits................. Vegetables...........
WEDNESDAY					Fat free Lowfat Milk dairy.............. Whole Grains
THURSDAY					Lean Meat Fish &Poultry............... Nut Seeds & Legumes..............
FRIDAY					Oils...................... Sweets Salt.......... Alcohol...............
SATURDAY					Gaols Success Base Planer Calories..................
SUNDAY					

1 Week DASH Diet Workbook...Calories

	Breakfast	Lunch	Dinner	Snacks	DASH Diet Base On............Calories
MONDAY					Note......................... ....
TUESDAY					Fruits................... Vegetables............
WEDNESDAY					Fat free Lowfat Milk dairy............... Whole Grains ....
THURSDAY					Lean Meat Fish &Poultry................ Nut Seeds & Legumes...............
FRIDAY					Oils....................... .... Sweets Salt.......... Alcohol................
SATURDAY					.... Gaols Success Base Planer Calories....................
SUNDAY					....

1 Week DASH Diet Workbook...Calories					
	Breakfast	Lunch	Dinner	Snacks	DASH Diet Base On..............Calories
MONDAY					Note.........................
TUESDAY					Fruits.................... Vegetables............
					Fat free Lowfat Milk dairy..............
WEDNESDAY					Whole Grains ....
THURSDAY					Lean Meat Fish &Poultry...............
					Nut Seeds & Legumes..............
FRIDAY					Oils....................... .... Sweets Salt.......... .... Alcohol................
SATURDAY					....
SUNDAY					Gaols Success Base Planer Calories................... ....

1 Week DASH Diet Workbook..Calories

	Breakfast	Lunch	Dinner	Snacks	DASH Diet Base On............Calories
MONDAY					Note..........................
TUESDAY					Fruits................... Vegetables............
WEDNESDAY					Fat free Lowfat Milk dairy............... Whole Grains
THURSDAY					Lean Meat Fish &Poultry............... Nut Seeds & Legumes...............
FRIDAY					Oils...................... Sweets Salt.......... Alcohol................
SATURDAY					
SUNDAY					Gaols Success Base Planer Calories....................

1 Week DASH Diet Workbook..Calories

	Breakfast	Lunch	Dinner	Snacks	DASH Diet
					Base On.............Calories
MONDAY					Note........................
TUESDAY					Fruits................... Vegetables............
					Fat free Lowfat Milk dairy..............
WEDNESDAY					Whole Grains
THURSDAY					Lean Meat Fish &Poultry...............
					Nut Seeds & Legumes..............
FRIDAY					Oils.....................
					Sweets Salt.......... Alcohol...............
SATURDAY					
					Gaols Success Base Planer Calories................
SUNDAY					

1 Week DASH Diet Workbook..Calories					
	Breakfast	Lunch	Dinner	Snacks	**DASH Diet** Base On............Calories
MONDAY					Note........................
TUESDAY					Fruits.................. Vegetables............
WEDNESDAY					Fat free Lowfat Milk dairy.............. Whole Grains ....
THURSDAY					Lean Meat Fish &Poultry................ Nut Seeds & Legumes..............
FRIDAY					Oils...................... .... Sweets Salt.......... .... Alcohol.................
SATURDAY					
SUNDAY					Gaols Success Base Planer Calories................... ....

1 Week DASH Diet Workbook..Calories

	Breakfast	Lunch	Dinner	Snacks	DASH Diet
					Base On............Calories
MONDAY					Note.........................
TUESDAY					Fruits................. Vegetables............
WEDNESDAY					Fat free Lowfat Milk dairy............. Whole Grains
THURSDAY					Lean Meat Fish &Poultry............... Nut Seeds & Legumes.............
FRIDAY					Oils.................... Sweets Salt......... Alcohol...............
SATURDAY					
SUNDAY					Gaols Success Base Planer Calories.................

1 Week DASH Diet Workbook..Calories					
	Breakfast	Lunch	Dinner	Snacks	DASH Diet Base On.............Calories
MONDAY					Note........................ ....
TUESDAY					Fruits................... Vegetables............
WEDNESDAY					Fat free Lowfat Milk dairy.............. Whole Grains ....
THURSDAY					Lean Meat Fish &Poultry................ Nut Seeds & Legumes..............
FRIDAY					Oils...................... .... Sweets Salt.......... .... Alcohol................
SATURDAY					....
SUNDAY					Gaols Success Base Planer Calories................... ....

1 Week DASH Diet Workbook...Calories

	Breakfast	Lunch	Dinner	Snacks	DASH Diet Base On............Calories
MONDAY					Note........................
TUESDAY					Fruits................. Vegetables............
WEDNESDAY					Fat free Lowfat Milk dairy.............. Whole Grains
THURSDAY					Lean Meat Fish &Poultry............... Nut Seeds & Legumes.............
FRIDAY					Oils.................... Sweets Salt......... Alcohol...............
SATURDAY					
SUNDAY					Gaols Success Base Planer Calories...................

1 Week DASH Diet Workbook..Calories				

	Breakfast	Lunch	Dinner	Snacks	DASH Diet Base On............Calories
MONDAY					Note........................ ....
TUESDAY					Fruits................. Vegetables............
					Fat free Lowfat Milk dairy..............
WEDNESDAY					Whole Grains ....
THURSDAY					Lean Meat Fish &Poultry................ Nut Seeds & Legumes...............
FRIDAY					Oils........................ .... Sweets Salt.......... .... Alcohol.................
SATURDAY					....
SUNDAY					**Gaols Success** Base Planer Calories.................... ....

1 Week DASH Diet Workbook..Calories

	Breakfast	Lunch	Dinner	Snacks	DASH Diet
					Base On............Calories
MONDAY					Note........................
TUESDAY					Fruits.................. Vegetables............
					Fat free Lowfat Milk dairy...............
WEDNESDAY					Whole Grains
THURSDAY					Lean Meat Fish &Poultry................ Nut Seeds & Legumes..............
FRIDAY					Oils..................... Sweets Salt.......... Alcohol................
SATURDAY					
SUNDAY					Gaols Success Base Planer Calories...................

1 Week DASH Diet Workbook..Calories

	Breakfast	Lunch	Dinner	Snacks	DASH Diet
MONDAY					Base On.............Calories Note........................
TUESDAY					Fruits................. Vegetables............
WEDNESDAY					Fat free Lowfat Milk dairy............. Whole Grains
THURSDAY					Lean Meat Fish &Poultry............... Nut Seeds & Legumes.............
FRIDAY					Oils..................... Sweets Salt.......... Alcohol...............
SATURDAY					
SUNDAY					Gaols Success Base Planer Calories..................

1 Week DASH Diet Workbook...Calories

	Breakfast	Lunch	Dinner	Snacks	DASH Diet Base On.............Calories
MONDAY					Note......................
TUESDAY					Fruits................. Vegetables............
WEDNESDAY					Fat free Lowfat Milk dairy............... Whole Grains ....
THURSDAY					Lean Meat Fish &Poultry................ Nut Seeds & Legumes..............
FRIDAY					Oils........................ .... Sweets Salt.......... .... Alcohol................
SATURDAY					.... **Gaols Success** Base Planer
SUNDAY					Calories.................... ....

	Breakfast	Lunch	Dinner	Snacks	DASH Diet
					Base On...........Calories
MONDAY					Note......................
TUESDAY					Fruits................. Vegetables...........
					Fat free Lowfat Milk dairy..............
WEDNESDAY					Whole Grains ....
THURSDAY					Lean Meat Fish &Poultry............... Nut Seeds & Legumes..............
FRIDAY					Oils..................... .... Sweets Salt.......... Alcohol...............
SATURDAY					
SUNDAY					Gaols Success Base Planer Calories.................

1 Week DASH Diet Workbook.......................................Calories

1 Week DASH Diet Workbook...Calories

	Breakfast	Lunch	Dinner	Snacks	DASH Diet Base On............Calories
MONDAY					Note........................
TUESDAY					Fruits................. Vegetables............
					Fat free Lowfat Milk dairy..............
WEDNESDAY					Whole Grains ....
THURSDAY					Lean Meat Fish &Poultry................
					Nut Seeds & Legumes..............
FRIDAY					Oils........................ ....
					Sweets Salt.......... Alcohol................
SATURDAY					
SUNDAY					Gaols Success Base Planer Calories..................

	Breakfast	Lunch	Dinner	Snacks	DASH Diet
					Base On.............Calories
MONDAY					Note........................ ....
TUESDAY					Fruits.................... Vegetables.............
					Fat free Lowfat Milk dairy..............
WEDNESDAY					Whole Grains ....
THURSDAY					Lean Meat Fish &Poultry................ Nut Seeds & Legumes...............
FRIDAY					Oils....................... .... Sweets Salt.......... .... Alcohol................
SATURDAY					.... **Gaols Success** Base Planer
SUNDAY					Calories................ ....

1 Week DASH Diet Workbook..Calories

1 Week DASH Diet Workbook...Calories

	Breakfast	Lunch	Dinner	Snacks	DASH Diet Base On............Calories
MONDAY					Note.........................
TUESDAY					Fruits.................... Vegetables............
WEDNESDAY					Fat free Lowfat Milk dairy............... Whole Grains ....
THURSDAY					Lean Meat Fish &Poultry................ Nut Seeds & Legumes..............
FRIDAY					Oils...................... .... Sweets Salt.......... Alcohol................
SATURDAY					 Gaols Success Base Planer Calories...................
SUNDAY					....

| 1 Week DASH Diet Workbook..Calories |

	Breakfast	Lunch	Dinner	Snacks	DASH Diet Base On............Calories
MONDAY					Note......................... ....
TUESDAY					Fruits................... Vegetables............
WEDNESDAY					Fat free Lowfat Milk dairy............... Whole Grains ....
THURSDAY					Lean Meat Fish &Poultry................ Nut Seeds & Legumes.............
FRIDAY					Oils...................... .... Sweets Salt.......... .... Alcohol................
SATURDAY					....
SUNDAY					Gaols Success Base Planer Calories................... ....

1 Week DASH Diet Workbook...Calories					
	Breakfast	Lunch	Dinner	Snacks	**DASH Diet** Base On............Calories
MONDAY					Note....................... ....
TUESDAY					Fruits................... Vegetables............
WEDNESDAY					Fat free Lowfat Milk dairy.............. Whole Grains ....
THURSDAY					Lean Meat Fish &Poultry............... Nut Seeds & Legumes..............
FRIDAY					Oils...................... .... Sweets Salt.......... .... Alcohol................
SATURDAY					....
SUNDAY					**Gaols Success** Base Planer Calories................... ....

1 Week DASH Diet Workbook...Calories

	Breakfast	Lunch	Dinner	Snacks	DASH Diet
					Base On............Calories
MONDAY					Note.......................
TUESDAY					Fruits................. Vegetables............
WEDNESDAY					Fat free Lowfat Milk dairy............... Whole Grains
THURSDAY					Lean Meat Fish &Poultry................ Nut Seeds & Legumes...............
FRIDAY					Oils....................... Sweets Salt.......... Alcohol................
SATURDAY					
SUNDAY					Gaols Success Base Planer Calories....................

1 Week DASH Diet Workbook...Calories

	Breakfast	Lunch	Dinner	Snacks	DASH Diet Base On............Calories
MONDAY					Note.........................
TUESDAY					Fruits.................. Vegetables............
WEDNESDAY					Fat free Lowfat Milk dairy.............. Whole Grains ....
THURSDAY					Lean Meat Fish &Poultry............... Nut Seeds & Legumes..............
FRIDAY					Oils....................... .... Sweets Salt.......... .... Alcohol................
SATURDAY					....
SUNDAY					Gaols Success Base Planer Calories................... ....

1 Week DASH Diet Workbook...Calories

	Breakfast	Lunch	Dinner	Snacks	DASH Diet Base On............Calories
MONDAY					Note........................
TUESDAY					Fruits................... Vegetables............
WEDNESDAY					Fat free Lowfat Milk dairy.............. Whole Grains
THURSDAY					Lean Meat Fish &Poultry............... Nut Seeds & Legumes..............
FRIDAY					Oils..................... Sweets Salt.......... Alcohol................
SATURDAY					
SUNDAY					Gaols Success Base Planer Calories....................

| 1 Week DASH Diet Workbook..Calories | | | | | |

	Breakfast	Lunch	Dinner	Snacks	DASH Diet
					Base On.............Calories
MONDAY					Note........................
TUESDAY					Fruits................... Vegetables............
					Fat free Lowfat Milk dairy..............
WEDNESDAY					Whole Grains ....
THURSDAY					Lean Meat Fish &Poultry.............. Nut Seeds & Legumes..............
FRIDAY					Oils...................... .... Sweets Salt.......... .... Alcohol................
SATURDAY					....
SUNDAY					Gaols Success Base Planer Calories................ ....

1 Week DASH Diet Workbook..Calories

	Breakfast	Lunch	Dinner	Snacks	DASH Diet Base On............Calories
MONDAY					Note......................... ....
TUESDAY					Fruits..................... Vegetables...........
WEDNESDAY					Fat free Lowfat Milk dairy...............
					Whole Grains ....
THURSDAY					Lean Meat Fish &Poultry................
					Nut Seeds & Legumes..............
FRIDAY					Oils..........................
					Sweets Salt.......... Alcohol.................
SATURDAY					....
SUNDAY					Gaols Success Base Planer Calories..................

1 Week DASH Diet Workbook...Calories

	Breakfast	Lunch	Dinner	Snacks	DASH Diet
					Base On.............Calories
MONDAY					Note.......................
TUESDAY					Fruits................... Vegetables............
WEDNESDAY					Fat free Lowfat Milk dairy.............. Whole Grains ....
THURSDAY					Lean Meat Fish &Poultry............... Nut Seeds & Legumes..............
FRIDAY					Oils...................... Sweets Salt.......... Alcohol................
SATURDAY					
SUNDAY					Gaols Success Base Planer Calories.................

1 Week DASH Diet Workbook...Calories

	Breakfast	Lunch	Dinner	Snacks	DASH Diet Base On............Calories
MONDAY					Note......................
TUESDAY					Fruits................. Vegetables............
WEDNESDAY					Fat free Lowfat Milk dairy.............. Whole Grains
THURSDAY					Lean Meat Fish &Poultry................ Nut Seeds & Legumes..............
FRIDAY					Oils...................... Sweets Salt.......... Alcohol................
SATURDAY					
SUNDAY					Gaols Success Base Planer Calories..................

1 Week DASH Diet Workbook..Calories

	Breakfast	Lunch	Dinner	Snacks	DASH Diet
					Base On.............Calories
MONDAY					Note........................
TUESDAY					Fruits................... Vegetables............
					Fat free Lowfat Milk dairy..............
WEDNESDAY					Whole Grains ....
THURSDAY					Lean Meat Fish &Poultry...............
					Nut Seeds & Legumes..............
FRIDAY					Oils.................... ....
					Sweets Salt.......... .... Alcohol................
SATURDAY					
SUNDAY					Gaols Success Base Planer Calories..................

1 Week DASH Diet Workbook..Calories

	Breakfast	Lunch	Dinner	Snacks	DASH Diet Base On............Calories
MONDAY					Note...................... ....
TUESDAY					Fruits................... Vegetables............
WEDNESDAY					Fat free Lowfat Milk dairy.............. Whole Grains ....
THURSDAY					Lean Meat Fish &Poultry............... Nut Seeds & Legumes..............
FRIDAY					Oils..................... .... Sweets Salt.......... .... Alcohol................
SATURDAY					....
SUNDAY					Gaols Success Base Planer Calories................... ....

1 Week DASH Diet Workbook..Calories					
	Breakfast	Lunch	Dinner	Snacks	**DASH Diet** Base On.............Calories
MONDAY					Note........................ Fruits.................... Vegetables............
TUESDAY					Fat free Lowfat Milk dairy..............
WEDNESDAY					Whole Grains
THURSDAY					Lean Meat Fish &Poultry............... Nut Seeds & Legumes..............
FRIDAY					Oils....................... Sweets Salt.......... Alcohol................
SATURDAY					
SUNDAY					**Gaols Success** Base Planer Calories...................

1 Week DASH Diet Workbook..Calories

	Breakfast	Lunch	Dinner	Snacks	DASH Diet Base On...........Calories
MONDAY					Note........................ ....
TUESDAY					Fruits.................. Vegetables............
WEDNESDAY					Fat free Lowfat Milk dairy.............. Whole Grains ....
THURSDAY					Lean Meat Fish &Poultry................ Nut Seeds & Legumes..............
FRIDAY					Oils..................... .... Sweets Salt.......... .... Alcohol................
SATURDAY					....
SUNDAY					Gaols Success Base Planer Calories................... ....

1 Week DASH Diet Workbook...Calories

	Breakfast	Lunch	Dinner	Snacks	DASH Diet Base On.............Calories
MONDAY					Note.......................
TUESDAY					Fruits.................. Vegetables............
WEDNESDAY					Fat free Lowfat Milk dairy.............. Whole Grains ....
THURSDAY					Lean Meat Fish &Poultry.............. Nut Seeds & Legumes.............
FRIDAY					Oils..................... .... Sweets Salt......... .... Alcohol...............
SATURDAY					....
SUNDAY					Gaols Success Base Planer Calories.................. ....

1 Week DASH Diet Workbook..Calories

	Breakfast	Lunch	Dinner	Snacks	DASH Diet Base On.............Calories
MONDAY					Note........................
TUESDAY					Fruits................. Vegetables............
WEDNESDAY					Fat free Lowfat Milk dairy............... Whole Grains
THURSDAY					Lean Meat Fish &Poultry................ Nut Seeds & Legumes...............
FRIDAY					Oils....................... Sweets Salt.......... Alcohol.................
SATURDAY					
SUNDAY					Gaols Success Base Planer Calories....................

1 Week DASH Diet Workbook...Calories

	Breakfast	Lunch	Dinner	Snacks	DASH Diet
					Base On............Calories
MONDAY					Note.........................
TUESDAY					Fruits.................... Vegetables............
WEDNESDAY					Fat free Lowfat Milk dairy.............. Whole Grains ....
THURSDAY					Lean Meat Fish &Poultry............... Nut Seeds & Legumes.............
FRIDAY					Oils.................... .... Sweets Salt.......... .... Alcohol................
SATURDAY					....
SUNDAY					**Gaols Success** Base Planer Calories..................

1 Week DASH Diet Workbook...Calories

	Breakfast	Lunch	Dinner	Snacks	DASH Diet
					Base On.............Calories
MONDAY					Note........................
TUESDAY					Fruits.................. Vegetables............
WEDNESDAY					Fat free Lowfat Milk dairy............... Whole Grains
THURSDAY					Lean Meat Fish &Poultry................ Nut Seeds & Legumes...............
FRIDAY					Oils...................... Sweets Salt........... Alcohol.................
SATURDAY					
SUNDAY					Gaols Success Base Planer Calories.................

1 Week DASH Diet Workbook...Calories					

	Breakfast	Lunch	Dinner	Snacks	DASH Diet Base On...........Calories
MONDAY					Note........................ ....
TUESDAY					**Fruits.................** **Vegetables...........**
WEDNESDAY					**Fat free Lowfat** **Milk dairy..............** **Whole Grains** ....
THURSDAY					**Lean Meat Fish** **&Poultry...............** **Nut Seeds** **& Legumes...............**
FRIDAY					**Oils......................** .... **Sweets Salt..........** .... **Alcohol................**
SATURDAY					.... **Gaols Success** Base Planer
SUNDAY					Calories.................... ....

1 Week DASH Diet Workbook..Calories

	Breakfast	Lunch	Dinner	Snacks	DASH Diet
					Base On............Calories
MONDAY					Note........................
TUESDAY					Fruits.................. Vegetables...........
					Fat free Lowfat Milk dairy..............
WEDNESDAY					Whole Grains ....
THURSDAY					Lean Meat Fish &Poultry............... Nut Seeds & Legumes.............
FRIDAY					Oils..................... Sweets Salt.......... Alcohol..............
SATURDAY					
SUNDAY					Gaols Success Base Planer Calories.................

	Breakfast	Lunch	Dinner	Snacks	DASH Diet
					Base On............Calories
MONDAY					Note...
TUESDAY					Fruits.................. Vegetables.............
WEDNESDAY					Fat free Lowfat Milk dairy............... Whole Grains ....
THURSDAY					Lean Meat Fish &Poultry................. Nut Seeds & Legumes...............
FRIDAY					Oils....................... .... Sweets Salt.......... .... Alcohol................
SATURDAY					....
SUNDAY					**Gaols Success** Base Planer Calories.................... ....

1 Week DASH Diet Workbook...Calories

1 Week DASH Diet Workbook...Calories

	Breakfast	Lunch	Dinner	Snacks	DASH Diet
					Base On............Calories
MONDAY					Note...................... ....
TUESDAY					Fruits.................. Vegetables...........
					Fat free Lowfat Milk dairy..............
WEDNESDAY					Whole Grains ....
THURSDAY					Lean Meat Fish &Poultry............... Nut Seeds & Legumes..............
FRIDAY					Oils...................... .... Sweets Salt.......... Alcohol................
SATURDAY					....
SUNDAY					**Gaols Success** Base Planer Calories.................... ....

	Breakfast	Lunch	Dinner	Snacks	DASH Diet
					Base On.............Calories
MONDAY					Note........................
TUESDAY					Fruits.................. Vegetables...........
					Fat free Lowfat Milk dairy..............
WEDNESDAY					Whole Grains
THURSDAY					Lean Meat Fish &Poultry................ Nut Seeds & Legumes..............
FRIDAY					Oils................... Sweets Salt.......... Alcohol................
SATURDAY					
SUNDAY					Gaols Success Base Planer Calories....................

1 Week DASH Diet Workbook...Calories

1 Week DASH Diet Workbook..Calories					

	Breakfast	Lunch	Dinner	Snacks	DASH Diet Base On............Calories
MONDAY					Note.........................
TUESDAY					Fruits................. Vegetables............
					Fat free Lowfat Milk dairy..............
WEDNESDAY					Whole Grains ....
THURSDAY					Lean Meat Fish &Poultry..............
					Nut Seeds & Legumes..............
FRIDAY					Oils....................... ....
					Sweets Salt.......... .... Alcohol................
SATURDAY					....
SUNDAY					Gaols Success Base Planer Calories.................... ....

1 Week DASH Diet Workbook..Calories

	Breakfast	Lunch	Dinner	Snacks	DASH Diet Base On.............Calories
MONDAY					Note........................ ....
TUESDAY					**Fruits...................** Vegetables............
					Fat free Lowfat Milk dairy..............
WEDNESDAY					**Whole Grains** ....
THURSDAY					**Lean Meat Fish** &Poultry...............
					Nut Seeds & Legumes..............
FRIDAY					Oils...................... ....
					Sweets Salt.......... .... Alcohol................
SATURDAY					....
					Gaols Success Base Planer
SUNDAY					Calories................... ....

	Breakfast	Lunch	Dinner	Snacks	DASH Diet
					Base On............Calories
MONDAY					Note.........................
TUESDAY					Fruits.................. Vegetables...........
WEDNESDAY					Fat free Lowfat Milk dairy.............. Whole Grains
THURSDAY					Lean Meat Fish &Poultry............... Nut Seeds & Legumes............
FRIDAY					Oils...................... Sweets Salt.......... Alcohol...............
SATURDAY					
SUNDAY					Gaols Success Base Planer Calories..................

1 Week DASH Diet Workbook..Calories

	Breakfast	Lunch	Dinner	Snacks	DASH Diet
					Base On............Calories
MONDAY					Note........................
TUESDAY					Fruits................. Vegetables............
WEDNESDAY					Fat free Lowfat Milk dairy.............. Whole Grains ....
THURSDAY					Lean Meat Fish &Poultry.............. Nut Seeds & Legumes..............
FRIDAY					Oils..................... .... Sweets Salt.......... Alcohol................
SATURDAY					
SUNDAY					Gaols Success Base Planer Calories................

1 Week DASH Diet Workbook...Calories

1 Week DASH Diet Workbook...Calories				

	Breakfast	Lunch	Dinner	Snacks	DASH Diet Base On.............Calories
MONDAY					Note........................ ....
TUESDAY					Fruits.................. Vegetables...........
WEDNESDAY					Fat free Lowfat Milk dairy............... Whole Grains ....
THURSDAY					Lean Meat Fish &Poultry................ Nut Seeds & Legumes..............
FRIDAY					Oils....................... .... Sweets Salt.......... .... Alcohol................
SATURDAY					
SUNDAY					Gaols Success Base Planer Calories.................... ....

1 Week DASH Diet Workbook...Calories

	Breakfast	Lunch	Dinner	Snacks	DASH Diet
					Base On.............Calories
MONDAY					Note........................
TUESDAY					Fruits.................. Vegetables.............
					Fat free Lowfat Milk dairy..............
WEDNESDAY					Whole Grains
THURSDAY					Lean Meat Fish &Poultry............... Nut Seeds & Legumes.............
FRIDAY					Oils...................... Sweets Salt......... Alcohol...............
SATURDAY					
SUNDAY					Gaols Success Base Planer Calories................

1 Week DASH Diet Workbook..Calories

	Breakfast	Lunch	Dinner	Snacks	DASH Diet Base On............Calories
MONDAY					Note......................
TUESDAY					Fruits................... Vegetables............ Fat free Lowfat Milk dairy..............
WEDNESDAY					Whole Grains
THURSDAY					Lean Meat Fish &Poultry................ Nut Seeds & Legumes..............
FRIDAY					Oils...................... Sweets Salt.......... Alcohol................
SATURDAY					
SUNDAY					Gaols Success Base Planer Calories................

1 Week DASH Diet Workbook..Calories				

	Breakfast	Lunch	Dinner	Snacks	DASH Diet Base On.............Calories
MONDAY					Note......................... ....
TUESDAY					Fruits.................. Vegetables............
					Fat free Lowfat Milk dairy..............
WEDNESDAY					Whole Grains ....
THURSDAY					Lean Meat Fish &Poultry.............. Nut Seeds & Legumes..............
FRIDAY					Oils...................... .... Sweets Salt.......... .... Alcohol................
SATURDAY					.... Gaols Success Base Planer Calories................
SUNDAY					....

1 Week DASH Diet Workbook...Calories					
	Breakfast	**Lunch**	**Dinner**	**Snacks**	**DASH Diet** Base On.............Calories
MONDAY					Note....................... ....
TUESDAY					Fruits..................... Vegetables............
					Fat free Lowfat Milk dairy...............
WEDNESDAY					Whole Grains ....
THURSDAY					Lean Meat Fish &Poultry................ Nut Seeds & Legumes..............
FRIDAY					Oils....................... .... Sweets Salt........... Alcohol.................
SATURDAY					....
SUNDAY					**Gaols Success** Base Planer Calories................... ....

1 Week DASH Diet Workbook...Calories

	Breakfast	Lunch	Dinner	Snacks	DASH Diet
					Base On.............Calories
MONDAY					Note....................
TUESDAY					Fruits.................. Vegetables............
					Fat free Lowfat Milk dairy..............
WEDNESDAY					Whole Grains ....
THURSDAY					Lean Meat Fish &Poultry............... Nut Seeds & Legumes..............
FRIDAY					Oils.................... .... Sweets Salt.......... .... Alcohol................
SATURDAY					....
SUNDAY					Gaols Success Base Planer Calories..................

1 Week DASH Diet Workbook...Calories

	Breakfast	Lunch	Dinner	Snacks	DASH Diet Base On............Calories
MONDAY					Note......................
TUESDAY					Fruits.................. Vegetables...........
WEDNESDAY					Fat free Lowfat Milk dairy.............. Whole Grains
THURSDAY					Lean Meat Fish &Poultry............... Nut Seeds & Legumes.............
FRIDAY					Oils...................... Sweets Salt.......... Alcohol...............
SATURDAY					
SUNDAY					Gaols Success Base Planer Calories..................

1 Week DASH Diet Workbook...Calories

	Breakfast	Lunch	Dinner	Snacks	DASH Diet Base On............Calories
MONDAY					Note............................
TUESDAY					Fruits.................. Vegetables............
WEDNESDAY					Fat free Lowfat Milk dairy.............. Whole Grains ....
THURSDAY					Lean Meat Fish &Poultry............... Nut Seeds & Legumes.............
FRIDAY					Oils..................... Sweets Salt......... Alcohol...............
SATURDAY					
SUNDAY					Gaols Success Base Planer Calories.................

1 Week DASH Diet Workbook..Calories					
	Breakfast	**Lunch**	**Dinner**	**Snacks**	**DASH Diet** Base On.............Calories
MONDAY					Note....................... ....
TUESDAY					Fruits................... Vegetables............
WEDNESDAY					Fat free Lowfat Milk dairy.............. Whole Grains ....
THURSDAY					Lean Meat Fish &Poultry................ Nut Seeds & Legumes...............
FRIDAY					Oils....................... .... Sweets Salt.......... .... Alcohol................
SATURDAY					....
SUNDAY					**Gaols Success** Base Planer Calories..................... ....

1 Week DASH Diet Workbook..Calories

	Breakfast	Lunch	Dinner	Snacks	DASH Diet Base On............Calories
MONDAY					Note.........................
TUESDAY					Fruits................. Vegetables............
WEDNESDAY					Fat free Lowfat Milk dairy............. Whole Grains
THURSDAY					Lean Meat Fish &Poultry............... Nut Seeds & Legumes...............
FRIDAY					Oils....................... Sweets Salt.......... Alcohol................
SATURDAY					Gaols Success Base Planer Calories.................
SUNDAY					

1 Week DASH Diet Workbook..Calories

	Breakfast	Lunch	Dinner	Snacks	DASH Diet Base On............Calories
MONDAY					Note........................
TUESDAY					Fruits................. Vegetables...........
WEDNESDAY					Fat free Lowfat Milk dairy............. Whole Grains
THURSDAY					Lean Meat Fish &Poultry............... Nut Seeds & Legumes..............
FRIDAY					Oils...................... Sweets Salt.......... Alcohol................
SATURDAY					
SUNDAY					Gaols Success Base Planer Calories..................

1 Week DASH Diet Workbook...Calories

	Breakfast	Lunch	Dinner	Snacks	DASH Diet Base On.............Calories
MONDAY					Note...................... ....
TUESDAY					Fruits................. Vegetables.............
					Fat free Lowfat Milk dairy..............
WEDNESDAY					Whole Grains ....
THURSDAY					Lean Meat Fish &Poultry..............
					Nut Seeds & Legumes..............
FRIDAY					Oils...................... ....
					Sweets Salt.......... .... Alcohol................
SATURDAY					....
SUNDAY					Gaols Success Base Planer Calories................... ....

1 Week DASH Diet Workbook..Calories

	Breakfast	Lunch	Dinner	Snacks	DASH Diet
					Base On.............Calories
MONDAY					Note........................ ....
TUESDAY					Fruits.................. Vegetables............
					Fat free Lowfat Milk dairy..............
WEDNESDAY					Whole Grains ....
THURSDAY					Lean Meat Fish &Poultry...............
					Nut Seeds & Legumes..............
FRIDAY					Oils...................... ....
					Sweets Salt.......... Alcohol...............
SATURDAY					....
SUNDAY					**Gaols Success** Base Planer Calories................. ....

	Breakfast	Lunch	Dinner	Snacks	DASH Diet
					Base On............Calories
MONDAY					Note..........................
TUESDAY					Fruits.................... Vegetables...........
WEDNESDAY					Fat free Lowfat Milk dairy.............. Whole Grains ....
THURSDAY					Lean Meat Fish &Poultry............... Nut Seeds & Legumes..............
FRIDAY					Oils..................... .... Sweets Salt.......... .... Alcohol................
SATURDAY					
SUNDAY					Gaols Success Base Planer Calories..................

1 Week DASH Diet Workbook...Calories

1 Week DASH Diet Workbook..Calories

	Breakfast	Lunch	Dinner	Snacks	DASH Diet
					Base On.............Calories
MONDAY					Note......................
TUESDAY					Fruits................... Vegetables...........
WEDNESDAY					Fat free Lowfat Milk dairy.............. Whole Grains ....
THURSDAY					Lean Meat Fish &Poultry............... Nut Seeds & Legumes..............
FRIDAY					Oils...................... .... Sweets Salt.......... .... Alcohol................
SATURDAY					
SUNDAY					Gaols Success Base Planer Calories................

1 Week DASH Diet Workbook...Calories

	Breakfast	Lunch	Dinner	Snacks	DASH Diet Base On............Calories
MONDAY					Note...................... ....
TUESDAY					Fruits.................. Vegetables...........
					Fat free Lowfat Milk dairy..............
WEDNESDAY					Whole Grains ....
THURSDAY					Lean Meat Fish &Poultry............... Nut Seeds & Legumes.............
FRIDAY					Oils...................... .... Sweets Salt.......... .... Alcohol................
SATURDAY					....
SUNDAY					Gaols Success Base Planer Calories................. ....

1 Week DASH Diet Workbook...Calories				

	Breakfast	Lunch	Dinner	Snacks	DASH Diet Base On............Calories
MONDAY					Note..................... ....
TUESDAY					Fruits................. Vegetables...........
WEDNESDAY					Fat free Lowfat Milk dairy.............. Whole Grains ....
THURSDAY					Lean Meat Fish &Poultry................ Nut Seeds & Legumes..............
FRIDAY					Oils...................... .... Sweets Salt.......... .... Alcohol.................
SATURDAY					....
SUNDAY					Gaols Success Base Planer Calories................... ....

1 Week DASH Diet Workbook...Calories

	Breakfast	Lunch	Dinner	Snacks	DASH Diet
MONDAY					Base On.............Calories Note........................
TUESDAY					Fruits................... Vegetables.............
					Fat free Lowfat Milk dairy..............
WEDNESDAY					Whole Grains ....
THURSDAY					Lean Meat Fish &Poultry............. Nut Seeds & Legumes..............
FRIDAY					Oils...................... ....
SATURDAY					Sweets Salt.......... .... Alcohol................
SUNDAY					Gaols Success Base Planer Calories.....................

1 Week DASH Diet Workbook...Calories

	Breakfast	Lunch	Dinner	Snacks	DASH Diet Base On............Calories
MONDAY					Note........................
TUESDAY					Fruits..................... Vegetables............
WEDNESDAY					Fat free Lowfat Milk dairy.............. Whole Grains
THURSDAY					Lean Meat Fish &Poultry................ Nut Seeds & Legumes...............
FRIDAY					Oils..................... Sweets Salt.......... Alcohol................
SATURDAY					
SUNDAY					Gaols Success Base Planer Calories....................

1 Week DASH Diet Workbook...Calories

	Breakfast	Lunch	Dinner	Snacks	DASH Diet
					Base On............Calories
MONDAY					Note........................
TUESDAY					Fruits................... Vegetables............
					Fat free Lowfat Milk dairy..............
WEDNESDAY					Whole Grains ....
THURSDAY					Lean Meat Fish &Poultry............... Nut Seeds & Legumes..............
FRIDAY					Oils..................... .... Sweets Salt.......... .... Alcohol................
SATURDAY					....
SUNDAY					Gaols Success Base Planer Calories...................

1 Week DASH Diet Workbook...Calories

	Breakfast	Lunch	Dinner	Snacks	DASH Diet Base On............Calories
MONDAY					Note........................ ....
TUESDAY					Fruits.................... Vegetables...........
					Fat free Lowfat Milk dairy..............
WEDNESDAY					Whole Grains ....
THURSDAY					Lean Meat Fish &Poultry............... Nut Seeds & Legumes..............
FRIDAY					Oils..................... .... Sweets Salt.......... .... Alcohol................
SATURDAY					....
SUNDAY					Gaols Success Base Planer Calories................ ....

1 Week DASH Diet Workbook...Calories

	Breakfast	Lunch	Dinner	Snacks	DASH Diet Base On..............Calories
MONDAY					Note...................... ....
TUESDAY					Fruits..................... Vegetables.............
WEDNESDAY					Fat free Lowfat Milk dairy.............. Whole Grains ....
THURSDAY					Lean Meat Fish &Poultry................ Nut Seeds & Legumes..............
FRIDAY					Oils....................... .... Sweets Salt.......... .... Alcohol................
SATURDAY					....
SUNDAY					Gaols Success Base Planer Calories................... ....

1 Week DASH Diet Workbook..Calories

	Breakfast	Lunch	Dinner	Snacks	DASH Diet Base On.............Calories
MONDAY					Note........................ ....
TUESDAY					Fruits................... Vegetables............
WEDNESDAY					Fat free Lowfat Milk dairy............... Whole Grains ....
THURSDAY					Lean Meat Fish &Poultry............... Nut Seeds & Legumes..............
FRIDAY					Oils....................... .... Sweets Salt.......... .... Alcohol................
SATURDAY					....
SUNDAY					Gaols Success Base Planer Calories................... ....

1 Week DASH Diet Workbook..Calories

	Breakfast	Lunch	Dinner	Snacks	DASH Diet Base On.............Calories
MONDAY					Note............................
TUESDAY					Fruits.................... Vegetables.............
WEDNESDAY					Fat free Lowfat Milk dairy............... Whole Grains
THURSDAY					Lean Meat Fish &Poultry............... Nut Seeds & Legumes...............
FRIDAY					Oils....................... Sweets Salt.......... Alcohol................
SATURDAY					
SUNDAY					Gaols Success Base Planer Calories....................

1 Week DASH Diet Workbook...Calories

	Breakfast	Lunch	Dinner	Snacks	DASH Diet
MONDAY					Base On.............Calories Note.......................
TUESDAY					Fruits.................... Vegetables............
WEDNESDAY					Fat free Lowfat Milk dairy.............. Whole Grains
THURSDAY					Lean Meat Fish &Poultry............... Nut Seeds & Legumes..............
FRIDAY					Oils..................... Sweets Salt......... Alcohol...............
SATURDAY					Gaols Success Base Planer
SUNDAY					Calories......................

1 Week DASH Diet Workbook...Calories

	Breakfast	Lunch	Dinner	Snacks	DASH Diet Base On.............Calories
MONDAY					Note......................... ....
TUESDAY					Fruits................... Vegetables.............
WEDNESDAY					Fat free Lowfat Milk dairy.............. Whole Grains ....
THURSDAY					Lean Meat Fish &Poultry............... Nut Seeds & Legumes...............
FRIDAY					Oils...................... .... Sweets Salt.......... Alcohol................
SATURDAY					....
SUNDAY					Gaols Success Base Planer Calories..................

1 Week DASH Diet Workbook...Calories					
	Breakfast	Lunch	Dinner	Snacks	DASH Diet Base On............Calories
MONDAY					Note....................... ....
TUESDAY					Fruits.................... Vegetables...........
WEDNESDAY					Fat free Lowfat Milk dairy.............. Whole Grains ....
THURSDAY					Lean Meat Fish &Poultry................ Nut Seeds & Legumes..............
FRIDAY					Oils...................... .... Sweets Salt.......... .... Alcohol................
SATURDAY					.... Gaols Success Base Planer
SUNDAY					Calories................... ....

1 Week DASH Diet Workbook...Calories

	Breakfast	Lunch	Dinner	Snacks	DASH Diet Base On.............Calories
MONDAY					Note....................... ....
TUESDAY					Fruits.................... Vegetables.............
WEDNESDAY					Fat free Lowfat Milk dairy............... Whole Grains ....
THURSDAY					Lean Meat Fish &Poultry............... Nut Seeds & Legumes..............
FRIDAY					Oils..................... .... Sweets Salt.......... .... Alcohol.................
SATURDAY					....
SUNDAY					Gaols Success Base Planer Calories.................... ....

1 Week DASH Diet Workbook...Calories

	Breakfast	Lunch	Dinner	Snacks	DASH Diet
					Base On.............Calories
MONDAY					Note.......................
TUESDAY					Fruits.............. Vegetables...........
WEDNESDAY					Fat free Lowfat Milk dairy.............. Whole Grains
THURSDAY					Lean Meat Fish &Poultry............... Nut Seeds & Legumes..............
FRIDAY					Oils..................... Sweets Salt.......... Alcohol...............
SATURDAY					Gaols Success Base Planer
SUNDAY					Calories...................

1 Week DASH Diet Workbook...Calories

	Breakfast	Lunch	Dinner	Snacks	DASH Diet Base On............Calories
MONDAY					Note..................... ....
TUESDAY					Fruits................... Vegetables............
WEDNESDAY					Fat free Lowfat Milk dairy............... Whole Grains ....
THURSDAY					Lean Meat Fish &Poultry............... Nut Seeds & Legumes...............
FRIDAY					Oils....................... .... Sweets Salt.......... .... Alcohol...............
SATURDAY					.... Gaols Success Base Planer
SUNDAY					Calories.................. ....

1 Week DASH Diet Workbook...Calories

	Breakfast	Lunch	Dinner	Snacks	DASH Diet Base On.............Calories
MONDAY					Note.......................
TUESDAY					Fruits................. Vegetables............
WEDNESDAY					Fat free Lowfat Milk dairy............... Whole Grains
THURSDAY					Lean Meat Fish &Poultry................ Nut Seeds & Legumes...............
FRIDAY					Oils..................... Sweets Salt.......... Alcohol................
SATURDAY					
SUNDAY					Gaols Success Base Planer Calories....................

1 Week DASH Diet Workbook..Calories				

	Breakfast	Lunch	Dinner	Snacks	DASH Diet Base On............Calories
MONDAY					Note.........................
TUESDAY					Fruits................... Vegetables............
WEDNESDAY					Fat free Lowfat Milk dairy............... Whole Grains ....
THURSDAY					Lean Meat Fish &Poultry............... Nut Seeds & Legumes..............
FRIDAY					Oils....................... .... Sweets Salt.......... .... Alcohol................
SATURDAY					.... Gaols Success Base Planer
SUNDAY					Calories................... ....

1 Week DASH Diet Workbook...Calories

	Breakfast	Lunch	Dinner	Snacks	DASH Diet Base On.............Calories
MONDAY					Note.....................
TUESDAY					Fruits................. Vegetables...........
WEDNESDAY					Fat free Lowfat Milk dairy............. Whole Grains
THURSDAY					Lean Meat Fish &Poultry............... Nut Seeds & Legumes.............
FRIDAY					Oils..................... Sweets Salt.......... Alcohol...............
SATURDAY					
SUNDAY					Gaols Success Base Planer Calories..................

1 Week DASH Diet Workbook...Calories

	Breakfast	Lunch	Dinner	Snacks	DASH Diet Base On............Calories
MONDAY					Note........................
TUESDAY					Fruits................... Vegetables............
WEDNESDAY					Fat free Lowfat Milk dairy.............. Whole Grains
THURSDAY					Lean Meat Fish &Poultry............... Nut Seeds & Legumes..............
FRIDAY					Oils...................... Sweets Salt.......... Alcohol...............
SATURDAY					
SUNDAY					Gaols Success Base Planer Calories..................

1 Week DASH Diet Workbook..Calories

	Breakfast	Lunch	Dinner	Snacks	DASH Diet Base On............Calories
MONDAY					Note......................
TUESDAY					Fruits............. Vegetables............
WEDNESDAY					Fat free Lowfat Milk dairy............... Whole Grains
THURSDAY					Lean Meat Fish &Poultry............... Nut Seeds & Legumes..............
FRIDAY					Oils...................... Sweets Salt......... Alcohol................
SATURDAY					
SUNDAY					Gaols Success Base Planer Calories..................

1 Week DASH Diet Workbook..Calories

	Breakfast	Lunch	Dinner	Snacks	DASH Diet Base On............Calories
MONDAY					Note....................... ....
TUESDAY					Fruits................... Vegetables............ Fat free Lowfat Milk dairy..............
WEDNESDAY					Whole Grains ....
THURSDAY					Lean Meat Fish &Poultry.............. Nut Seeds & Legumes..............
FRIDAY					Oils..................... .... Sweets Salt.......... .... Alcohol................
SATURDAY					.... Gaols Success Base Planer
SUNDAY					Calories................... ....

1 Week DASH Diet Workbook..Calories

	Breakfast	Lunch	Dinner	Snacks	DASH Diet Base On............Calories
MONDAY					Note........................
TUESDAY					Fruits................... Vegetables...........
WEDNESDAY					Fat free Lowfat Milk dairy.............. Whole Grains ....
THURSDAY					Lean Meat Fish &Poultry............... Nut Seeds & Legumes.............
FRIDAY					Oils....................... .... Sweets Salt.......... Alcohol................
SATURDAY					....
SUNDAY					Gaols Success Base Planer Calories.................. ....

1 Week DASH Diet Workbook...Calories

	Breakfast	Lunch	Dinner	Snacks	DASH Diet
					Base On.............Calories
MONDAY					Note........................
TUESDAY					Fruits................. Vegetables...........
WEDNESDAY					Fat free Lowfat Milk dairy.............. Whole Grains ....
THURSDAY					Lean Meat Fish &Poultry.............. Nut Seeds & Legumes..............
FRIDAY					Oils..................... .... Sweets Salt.......... Alcohol...............
SATURDAY					
SUNDAY					Gaols Success Base Planer Calories..................

1 Week DASH Diet Workbook...Calories

	Breakfast	Lunch	Dinner	Snacks	DASH Diet Base On.............Calories
MONDAY					Note........................ ....
TUESDAY					Fruits................. Vegetables............
					Fat free Lowfat Milk dairy..............
WEDNESDAY					Whole Grains ....
THURSDAY					Lean Meat Fish &Poultry................ Nut Seeds & Legumes..............
FRIDAY					Oils..................... .... Sweets Salt.......... .... Alcohol................
SATURDAY					....
SUNDAY					Gaols Success Base Planer Calories.................... ....

1 Week DASH Diet Workbook..Calories

	Breakfast	Lunch	Dinner	Snacks	DASH Diet Base On.............Calories
MONDAY					Note........................
TUESDAY					Fruits................... Vegetables............ Fat free Lowfat Milk dairy..............
WEDNESDAY					Whole Grains ....
THURSDAY					Lean Meat Fish &Poultry............... Nut Seeds & Legumes..............
FRIDAY					Oils....................... .... Sweets Salt.......... .... Alcohol................
SATURDAY					....
SUNDAY					Gaols Success Base Planer Calories................... ....

1 Week DASH Diet Workbook...Calories				

	Breakfast	Lunch	Dinner	Snacks	DASH Diet Base On............Calories
MONDAY					Note......................... ....
TUESDAY					Fruits.................. Vegetables............
WEDNESDAY					Fat free Lowfat Milk dairy............... Whole Grains ....
THURSDAY					Lean Meat Fish &Poultry............... Nut Seeds & Legumes...............
FRIDAY					Oils....................... .... Sweets Salt.......... .... Alcohol................
SATURDAY					.... Gaols Success Base Planer
SUNDAY					Calories.................... ....

1 Week DASH Diet Workbook..Calories				
	Breakfast	Lunch	Dinner	Snacks	**DASH Diet** Base On.............Calories
MONDAY					Note.................... ....
TUESDAY					Fruits................... Vegetables............
WEDNESDAY					Fat free Lowfat Milk dairy.............. Whole Grains ....
THURSDAY					Lean Meat Fish &Poultry.............. Nut Seeds & Legumes..............
FRIDAY					Oils....................... .... Sweets Salt.......... .... Alcohol................
SATURDAY					....
SUNDAY					**Gaols Success** Base Planer Calories.................... ....

1 Week DASH Diet Workbook..Calories

	Breakfast	Lunch	Dinner	Snacks	DASH Diet Base On...........Calories
MONDAY					Note.......................
TUESDAY					Fruits................. Vegetables............
WEDNESDAY					Fat free Lowfat Milk dairy.............. Whole Grains
THURSDAY					Lean Meat Fish &Poultry............... Nut Seeds & Legumes..............
FRIDAY					Oils...................... Sweets Salt.......... Alcohol................
SATURDAY					Gaols Success Base Planer Calories...................
SUNDAY					

1 Week DASH Diet Workbook...Calories

	Breakfast	Lunch	Dinner	Snacks	DASH Diet Base On.............Calories
MONDAY					Note........................ ....
TUESDAY					Fruits................... Vegetables............
					Fat free Lowfat Milk dairy..............
WEDNESDAY					Whole Grains ....
THURSDAY					Lean Meat Fish &Poultry............... Nut Seeds & Legumes..............
FRIDAY					Oils...................... .... Sweets Salt.......... .... Alcohol................
SATURDAY					.... Gaols Success Base Planer Calories..................
SUNDAY					....

1 Week DASH Diet Workbook..Calories

	Breakfast	Lunch	Dinner	Snacks	DASH Diet Base On............Calories
MONDAY					Note........................ ....
TUESDAY					Fruits.................... Vegetables............
					Fat free Lowfat Milk dairy..............
WEDNESDAY					Whole Grains ....
THURSDAY					Lean Meat Fish &Poultry................ Nut Seeds & Legumes..............
FRIDAY					Oils....................... .... Sweets Salt.......... .... Alcohol................
SATURDAY					....
SUNDAY					Gaols Success Base Planer Calories................... ....

1 Week DASH Diet Workbook...Calories

	Breakfast	Lunch	Dinner	Snacks	DASH Diet Base On..............Calories
MONDAY					Note........................ Fruits.................. Vegetables............
TUESDAY					Fat free Lowfat Milk dairy..............
WEDNESDAY					Whole Grains ....
THURSDAY					Lean Meat Fish &Poultry............... Nut Seeds & Legumes..............
FRIDAY					Oils..................... .... Sweets Salt.......... Alcohol...............
SATURDAY					
SUNDAY					Gaols Success Base Planer Calories...................

1 Week DASH Diet Workbook..Calories

	Breakfast	Lunch	Dinner	Snacks	DASH Diet Base On.............Calories
MONDAY					Note........................
TUESDAY					Fruits.................... Vegetables...........
WEDNESDAY					Fat free Lowfat Milk dairy............... Whole Grains
THURSDAY					Lean Meat Fish &Poultry................ Nut Seeds & Legumes.............
FRIDAY					Oils...................... Sweets Salt.......... Alcohol................
SATURDAY					
SUNDAY					Gaols Success Base Planer Calories...................

1 Week DASH Diet Workbook...Calories

	Breakfast	Lunch	Dinner	Snacks	DASH Diet Base On............Calories
MONDAY					Note........................ ....
TUESDAY					Fruits................. Vegetables.............
WEDNESDAY					Fat free Lowfat Milk dairy.............. Whole Grains ....
THURSDAY					Lean Meat Fish &Poultry............... Nut Seeds & Legumes..............
FRIDAY					Oils....................... .... Sweets Salt.......... .... Alcohol................
SATURDAY					.... Gaols Success Base Planer
SUNDAY					Calories................... ....

1 Week DASH Diet Workbook..Calories

	Breakfast	Lunch	Dinner	Snacks	DASH Diet Base On............Calories
MONDAY					Note........................ ....
TUESDAY					Fruits................. Vegetables...........
WEDNESDAY					Fat free Lowfat Milk dairy.............. Whole Grains ....
THURSDAY					Lean Meat Fish &Poultry............... Nut Seeds & Legumes..............
FRIDAY					Oils....................... .... Sweets Salt.......... .... Alcohol................
SATURDAY					....
SUNDAY					Gaols Success Base Planer Calories................... ....

1 Week DASH Diet Workbook..Calories

	Breakfast	Lunch	Dinner	Snacks	DASH Diet Base On............Calories
MONDAY					Note......................
TUESDAY					Fruits................. Vegetables...........
WEDNESDAY					Fat free Lowfat Milk dairy.............. Whole Grains
THURSDAY					Lean Meat Fish &Poultry............... Nut Seeds & Legumes..............
FRIDAY					Oils...................... Sweets Salt.......... Alcohol...............
SATURDAY					Gaols Success Base Planer
SUNDAY					Calories..................

	Breakfast	Lunch	Dinner	Snacks	DASH Diet Base On............Calories
					Note........................ ....
MONDAY					
TUESDAY					Fruits.................. Vegetables...........
					Fat free Lowfat Milk dairy..............
WEDNESDAY					Whole Grains ....
THURSDAY					Lean Meat Fish &Poultry................ Nut Seeds & Legumes..............
FRIDAY					Oils....................... .... Sweets Salt.......... .... Alcohol................
SATURDAY					....
SUNDAY					Gaols Success Base Planer Calories................... ....

1 Week DASH Diet Workbook..Calories

1 Week DASH Diet Workbook...Calories

	Breakfast	Lunch	Dinner	Snacks	DASH Diet Base On.............Calories
MONDAY					Note...................... DASH Diet items below
TUESDAY					Fruits.................. Vegetables............
					Fat free Lowfat Milk dairy..............
WEDNESDAY					Whole Grains ....
THURSDAY					Lean Meat Fish &Poultry................ Nut Seeds & Legumes..............
FRIDAY					Oils...................... .... Sweets Salt.......... .... Alcohol................
SATURDAY					.... Gaols Success Base Planer
SUNDAY					Calories................... ....

1 Week DASH Diet Workbook...Calories					
	Breakfast	**Lunch**	**Dinner**	**Snacks**	**DASH Diet** Base On..............Calories
MONDAY					Note........................ ....
TUESDAY					Fruits.................... Vegetables............
					Fat free Lowfat Milk dairy.............
WEDNESDAY					Whole Grains ....
THURSDAY					Lean Meat Fish &Poultry................ Nut Seeds & Legumes..............
FRIDAY					Oils....................... .... Sweets Salt.......... .... Alcohol................
SATURDAY					....
SUNDAY					**Gaols Success** Base Planer Calories.................. ....

9 781982 010386